There's Light at the End of the Tunnel

Andrew Aldred

chipmunkapublishing
the mental health publisher

Andrew Aldred

All rights reserved, no part of this publication may be reproduced by any means, electronic, mechanical photocopying, documentary, film or in any other format without prior written permission of the publisher.

>Published by
>Chipmunkapublishing
>United Kingdom

http://www.chipmunkapublishing.com

Copyright © **Andrew Aldred 2017**

ISBN   978-1-78382-375-8

There's Light at the End of the Tunnel

Keeping Afloat

We're trying to keep each other afloat
But we're both beginning to tire
Thirty years of mental illness apiece
Her recent pneumonia and heart attack
And my diagnosis of throat cancer
The alcohol problem that resulted in our divorce
As soon as we've solved one problem
There's another two or three to take its place
Life's hard and relentless
We've still got each other
Our parents are refusing to die
And we're just as stubborn
But we're all in deep water
And none of us will float forever

Andrew Aldred

Bleeding me Dry

I tried to cut the cost of my television package recently
It cost me a hundred pounds for the telephone bill
To pay to get my package removed
I will still save a small amount of money
But surely these people are there to provide a service?
All they seem to want to do is sell me things that I don't want
I'm not here to pay for Rupert Murdoch's standard of living
Out of my paltry wage as an ex-soldier
They can get rid of cable television and the internet for me
I think we'd all be better off without it
The internet is a gigantic marketing machine to make money
Out of the gullible and impressionable people who use it
They offer us entertainment to take money off our hands
Things were better in the seventies
If you had four channels to watch
At least you knew what was on
The license fee was worth paying
At least we had the BBC
I don't know if they'll do away with that
These people running the media are so irresponsible
And they're doing their best to bleed me dry

There's Light at the End of the Tunnel

Cancer Treatment

I'd like having cancer a lot better
If it didn't involve travelling with a set of morons
Who seem intent on hating me
For having cancer at the same time as them
I can't say a right word in the taxi
And I'm always travelling with the same mad couple
God knows what they've got against me
I guess I'll just exercise the right to be wrong
They'll have to complain if they want to get rid of me
And then there's the driver who fancies my partner
I could be dying of cancer
But please don't take the only person I know away
Give me a break Mr Patel
And get a life of your own
Three more weeks to go
I hope I can see this through

Andrew Aldred

Corrupt World

I watched a program about the jails in Haiti today
They're not too different from our own
Just more overcrowded, dirty and disease ridden
Run by a bunch of immoral, inhuman beings
Who for some desperate reason want to work there
 They have no moral standards and ideas above their station
They're totally useless and all they want is money
Then by all means give them a job
They will be easy to control and manipulate
Because they have as many faults as the people they work for

There's Light at the End of the Tunnel

Congratulations

Congratulations, America!
On voting in your new president
The most corrupt and unscrupulous man in America
And also one of the richest
Put him in charge
Don't worry about healthcare
Don't worry about the poor
If you're white and rich
You'll be alright
If you're not you can die
Making Donald Trump richer
Or building a Mexican wall
Don't worry about riots
Or civil unrest
You voted him in
Give yourselves a round of applause
I'm sure the world is a better place!

Andrew Aldred

They're Killing me Again

People are trying to put me in my grave
It seems that they want to do it sooner
I want to wait a little while yet
I don't know what the solution is
Not drugs, alcohol, or cigarettes this time
The doctor says he'll cure my cancer
It seems to be up to me
To cure the general public of their disease
But I don't even know what they want
The world would like me to move on
From my semi-detached house
They don't like me paying the mortgage
Off handouts and treatment for cancer
I would like to give more to society
But I can only stretch so far
I'm old, tired and weakened
Hiding out with my woman
I've got races to win but I'm an old nag
I'd like to keep going forever
But sooner or later I'm going to collapse

There's Light at the End of the Tunnel

The Death of Cancer

The last remaining cancer cells are fighting
To stay alive inside my throat
As I fight to eat and sleep
And kill them off as they persevere
Clinging on like limpets to the hull of a ship
As the sleeping giant becomes a fugitive
Slowly and surely a victor will emerge
And I'm betting I can kill cancer this time

Andrew Aldred

Make an Example of Him

Donald Trump has got his chosen job
And everyone has started complaining
He's oblivious to Russian computer hacking
People are denouncing him as their president
Older statesmen are already keeping him in line
And although he is sat at the heart of his country
He will find it far from a license to do what he likes
He is going to be forced to do what is right
And forced to do what the people want
His dream job might turn out to be a nightmare
He will be a better person after his term
Or he will be dead
He will have to justify his election
Or America will make an example of him

There's Light at the End of the Tunnel

Separation

Some things are hard to get used to
Saying goodnight and going home
Breaks her heart and mine every night
Living in two different homes
No longer married but still in love
We've sacrificed such a lot to be together
At least now our relationship is working
It's difficult being separated
But harder being married and under the same roof

Andrew Aldred

One Nation One People

There's too many factions in modern society
There has been for centuries
If we could ever unite under one banner
As one nation and one people
It would sort out all the problems
There would be no need for war
There would be enough food for everyone
Everybody could get a fair deal
And no-one would be left behind
We're all at war with each other
If it's not the neighbours doing you in
It's the police or the department of work and pensions
Or your place of work
They all want to single somebody out
They pick on the disabled and the weak
Separate out the minorities to take the blame
To keep the rest of society satisfied
It's all so wrong and so stupid
We should be building bridges instead of burning them
We celebrate our differences but not our similarities
Will anything bring us all together?

There's Light at the End of the Tunnel

Blown Out and Humiliated

Britain and America have been to war
Many times over the past few years
We've been heavily involved in Iraq and Afghanistan
We're standing off in Syria
The Russians are taking centre stage
Sending warships through the English Channel
On the way to Aleppo
Was there no other way they could have gone?
It's all very crushing
Boris Johnson is trying to get the Anti-War people
To campaign outside the Russian Embassy
But it's all one big publicity stunt
We're not going to blow a Russian aircraft carrier out of the water
We might not have a base for out nuclear submarines
If Nicola Sturgeon and the SNP have their way
We've opted out of Europe
We're becoming increasingly small, weak and isolated
We've spent far too much money fighting wars recently
We don't want to argue with Russia
America is helping deal with ISIS in Iraq
Russia is backing Assad in Syria
We aren't needed there any more
Britain is not so great any more

Andrew Aldred

Christie Hospital

Here it is on the other side of Manchester
A hospital entirely dedicated to the treatment of cancer
I've been told I stand a very good chance
Of living through the next five years
Provided I give up smoking
Which doesn't seem such a difficult thing to do
When your existence is called into question
The nurses are bossy
I fainted the other day
But they've seen it all before
I've got a month of treatment in this wretched place
And I will get through it any way I can
How bad can it be?
Not much worse than it's been already
Twenty days of "must do" treatment
Will save my life for another time
I can die any time I like
But right now I want to carry on living

There's Light at the End of the Tunnel

Shut Him Up

The leader of the house of commons
Pulled a great stunt today
By saying Donald Trump would not get an audience there
That's one up the arse for the prime minister
She has just gone over to make a trade deal with him
The queen wants to see him
But is he really welcome in our country?
With his racist, woman-hating views on life
A lot of people have made it clear that he isn't
God bless you all! Is this fake news!
Is he actually going to come to England at all?
Or will he just stay in his own country?
Where for some bizarre reason he got voted in
A lot of people are telling him to shut up!

Andrew Aldred

Fake News

It's on television tonight
An entire program of "fake news"
Entertainment based on bullshit
In the middle there's an advert
For a television series
Called "When Fake News Was Funny"
And once it was!
In the days of the Daily Sport
Sadly I think we have progressed too far for that
Anything Donald Trump does not agree with is "fake news"
He has cornered the market!
Does anyone in America think he's doing anything good?
But looking back, was Tony Blair just as bad?
Going to war with Iraq over a set of lies
What will be Tony Blair's legacy?
Does anyone believe anything any more?
Is the whole world just an entertainment industry
For a set of facetious people sat in their armchairs?
When will we all get ourselves in check?
I don't know! Give me something real!

There's Light at the End of the Tunnel

The Meeting

It's a very mixed bunch of people
In this lecture room today
We get the introductions and do the icebreakers
And I try to talk to the woman next to me
About my life and how things are
And I try to listen to her
As she tells me everything is worse for somebody else
I know I'm emotionally strung out
And I've just raised the level of my psychiatric medication
And that the rest of the people on my table
Are secure in their careers and their middle-class life
We somehow find a way forward
Get our tasks done and show them to the group
And we discuss our slogan for the day
For this we choose "Make a Difference"
But has it made a difference to me?
As I thank the woman next to me
For allowing me to open up about my life
All its done is pass a couple of hours on
For me there is no difference
Nothing relevant, new or life-changing
Just the end of another meeting for the NHS

Andrew Aldred

What's up, Donald?

I'm watching the news closely, these days
And Donald Trump is never far away
He'll be building his Mexican wall
Restricting access to America
For all Muslims and foreigners
What's next? A war with China?
Is he going over to Russia to party with Alexander Putin
He's just been seen holding hands with Theresa May
Does anyone ever stop to think?
That maybe things were better under Obama
Has the world really gone crazy?
So I'll turn my television on tomorrow
And wonder what Trump is up to
What sweeping changes he is going to make
As he signs away people's rights and lives
Always in full public view
Is this what America wants?
If Donald Trump doesn't get himself killed
It's not looking good for everyone else

There's Light at the End of the Tunnel

No Redeeming Qualities

If I ever get myself into trouble
I'm old enough to know
I'll have to face the consequences
The cavalry won't be coming
And I'll have to dig myself out of the situation
When you're a man in his fifties
You have very few excuses
And very few redeeming qualities
Who you know is limited to your family
And maybe one or two friends
If you're lucky enough to have any
Ever since I was a child
It's always been my fault
I've always been to blame
Nobody is going to feel sorry for me
I'm a man in his fifties
And I have very few redeeming qualities

Andrew Aldred

Maggie's Army

It's thirty years on from Margaret Thatcher now
But her legacy lives on
I couldn't get a decent job if I was fit to do one
And there are plenty like me from our lost generation
The people who have done all the shit jobs
Who didn't get on after leaving school
I joined the army because I couldn't do anything else
And they've moved me from pillar to post ever since
Because after three short years I wasn't fit to serve
I've been judged mentally ill ever since
Because this is the best deal society will give me
All the decent jobs go to somebody else
I'm one of Thatcher's soldiers thirty years after the war

There's Light at the End of the Tunnel

Family Politics

If you're trying to get on with family
You've got to realise
That you're dealing with a bunch of people
Far more difficult to get on with
Than your average politicians
They all have their own character
Their own agenda
And their own personality
And they will only take so much off you
Which makes it very difficult
To get anything done at all
But if you ignore their faults
They might forgive you for yours
And if you give them something
They will give you something back
We all have our differences
And our own special allies
But if we do our best to get on
And shelve the politics for some other time

Andrew Aldred

Haters

I had to put something on Facebook the other day
I thought it was about time I said something
About my current situation
It was nothing out of the ordinary or offensive
But I got the wrong reaction
There's people with a lot less than myself out there
But they have to realise that's not my fault
My life could be cut short at any minute
I could suddenly wind up with nothing
People should be satisfied with their lot
Just like I have to be satisfied with mine
My situation is far from perfect
But it's really not that bad
Please don't make things any worse or harder for me
And I'll try my best not to hurt or offend
I've been hated enough all of my life
Get on with hating somebody else
I never intended to rattle anybody's cage

There's Light at the End of the Tunnel

Fear of Dying

I could worry myself silly every day
With the fear that my cancer might return
I could go to the doctor with every little complaint
In the vain hope of living forever
But it wouldn't do me any good
I'll just get on with living the best I can
I probably won't be dead today or tomorrow
And the day after that will take care of itself
I'd rather die a quick and painless death
Than live in agony and fear of dying
I'll just have to see what happens
But I'm not going to live in paranoia city
I've spent enough time there already

Andrew Aldred

Brexit

We are leaving the rest of Europe in the lurch
And they are getting a huge golden handshake off us
If Germany wants to carry the debt of the rest of Europe
In order to have a common currency
We've left them on their own to get on with it
They've got Europe in their pocket without fighting a war
Will they all face economic collapse?
We will not be around to face it with them
Britain will sink or swim on its own

There's Light at the End of the Tunnel

Consolation

Her mother is slowly dying
And so are my parents
She could have another heart attack
My cancer could have a resurgence
Her daughter is short of money
And the rest of the family have their problems
But we both have a small and considerable consolation
In that we both have each other
If she left I'm sure I wouldn't last forever
I might as well start smoking and drinking again
A life without love and friendship
Would be very hard to contemplate
She's still here and so am I

Andrew Aldred

Car-nage

I saw it on the news today
A Muslim man in a hire car
Charging up a pavement to parliament
Mowing down pedestrians
Stabbing a policeman
What has he achieved?
What were his reasons?
ISIS have claimed responsibility
Well I suppose they would
Half this man's family are in police custody
He had a girlfriend
Surely he had something to live for?
The British nationalists were on TV last night
I know life gets harder in middle age
At least this man is now dead
Which is very little consolation for his victims
What was he so furious about?
Most of the people he ran over were on holiday
I wish he'd got up on the right side of the bed

There's Light at the End of the Tunnel

Tied up and Free at the Same Time

We've got a house each to live in now
Although we spend most of our time together
And we'd be fools to leave the security
Of each having our own front door
Somehow it's brought us together
We're trying to take care of the family
Neither of us wants to mess around
Or bring other people into the relationship
We've sorted out our lifestyle
We've come a hell of a long way
Could we ever remarry?
Certainly not at this moment in time
We're getting on so well
Because we're not treading on each other's toes
Being married was a fantastic thing
But the marriage we had didn't suit us
You can lose your identity in a marriage
Everyone needs some space sometimes

Andrew Aldred

Rap Stars of Hollywood

How can these people fit all their egos in one room?
The answer is with difficulty and not for very long
Someone will lose their temper and storm off
Or do their best to knock somebody's block off
It's all good entertainment if you like that sort of thing
But which side of the fence are you on?
Do you admire the bloke with half a dozen girlfriends?
Would you like to drink champagne while you get your nails done?
Some of us would sell our souls for a life like this
Some of us are a bit older and realise it doesn't last forever
Souldja boy might as well enjoy his twenty fourth birthday
How many more will he have? He's totally wasted!
Do they make you sick with their wigs and their plumped-up lips?
Are they all so vulgar and trashy they're really ugly?
There's a certain fascination, but if you've seen one episode
The rest of them are going to be very much the same
It's reality TV at its best and worst all at the same time!

There's Light at the End of the Tunnel

American Bullshit

Who knows what is really going on in America at the moment?
Everyone is desperate for change. That's for sure.
They've got a maverick president who thinks he'll do what he wants
The Russians have influenced their general election
I'm not at all sure about this. Is it just an excuse for the chaos?
Is it a divided society that's falling apart? I think so.
It all seems to be a smokescreen. What will emerge?
When will we get some real news?
Is scaremongering all that's going on?
Will Donald Trump deliver on his Mexican wall?
Are the Russians really a subversive influence?
Should the world really be worried?
Everyone is sick of the fake news and the bullshit
Is reality too much to contemplate?

Andrew Aldred

Avatar

I saw a repeat of the film Avatar on TV last night
It's a very emotive film with a lot of current issues
For a start there's the environmental one
Where the government is destroying the forest for minerals
Just like we are destroying the rainforests
Capitalism versus mother nature on a grand scale
Then there's the hatred of the military and the job they do
Walking roughshod over people's lives for some greater good
There's a disabled man who is capable of being a hero
With the aid of technology and friendship
And the army general who wants to destroy everything
And isn't happy until he sees it all go up in smoke
There's the ancient ways of the tribal people
Who are on morally higher ground than the invaders
How do we hold onto our old ways and progress?
In these days of immorality and greed
Donald Trump didn't win the election of his environmental policies
There's no easy way to build a better world
But this is the highest grossing film of all time
So where the hell is the world going wrong?

There's Light at the End of the Tunnel

Drugs Epidemic

They are on the streets in Manchester today
Bodies in suspended animation
In weird positions on littered streets
They should know better but they don't
All they want to do is get out of their heads
It's like "Shaun of the dead" but it's not funny
They all look as if they are homeless
The clothes they are wearing give them away
This is what the boom in spice has given us
More work for the emergency services
People want to make the drug for themselves
And sell it on the street. This is the result.
The government has taken away legal highs
People are taking things into their own hands

Andrew Aldred

You can do whatever you want

The sky's the limit! Everything is achievable!
This is what you were taught at school
It's alright as long as you want to work in a factory
That's about the best you'll get these days
We can't all be singers, TV stars and athletes
It takes a hell of a lot of finance
And a great deal of effort and talent
What do you do if you're not that capable
Especially if you've got a burning ambition
To have a lifestyle and live like the rich
The best thing I ever achieved was to be a soldier
Some people don't even get that
You can do whatever you want
But only if you're a bloody celebrity

There's Light at the End of the Tunnel

Will you save us?

Donald Trump has sent his message to North Korea
And signed it on behalf of his country
He has strategically intervened in Syria
And narrowly avoided confrontation with the Russians
Does he want to use his nuclear arsenal?
Are himself and everyone else sick of diplomacy?
Is Donald Trump a hero or a villain?
Is he a warmonger or a bringer of peace?
Will he cure his country's sick economy?
Can he save us all or even himself?
Only time will tell. I'd love Donald Trump to be a great president
I'd love him to clear up the mess in Syria
I'd love him to neutralise North Korea
Will you save us, Mr Trump? Can you be a great president?

Andrew Aldred

My Heart's in the right place

You know you're going to have to trust me
And I'm going to have to trust you
You can't be in charge of me
Any more than I can be in charge of you
Everything has to be by mutual consent
Forget all your womanly wiles
They're a waste of time and so tedious
And I'll try to forget my pride
And get on with the job in hand
I'd like to think my heart is in the right place
But it's always going to need some company there

There's Light at the End of the Tunnel

Escalation of War

North Korea threatened a nuclear strike today
Do they really think they're invincible?
Do they really want to threaten Donald Trump?
It seems they do and they want a nuclear war
Do they care so little about their own people?
And the Americans they want to attack?
They're putting America in a very embarrassing situation
They can't back down. Will China step in?
North Korea and America!   It's all kicking off!

Andrew Aldred

Small-minded

He was selling mobile phones in a town centre shop
I was his last customer on a Friday afternoon
As he was serving me he got progressively more nervous
It was almost as if he was withdrawing from drugs
He was so desperate to get out of the shop
He deleted all the numbers on my sim card
And then all the numbers on my phone
Making everything impossible to retrieve
There was no apology at all, just an insistence
That it was nothing to do with him and all the fault of my old phone
I'll have to fill in the customer service review tomorrow
And he's going to get zero out of ten for everything
And a text message to EE about his poor service
Why do some people even bother to go to work?
I hope this small-minded young man finds something else to do
And I can get served by someone who wants to be there next time

There's Light at the End of the Tunnel

Power Struggle

We've got the United States of Germany
Trying to take over the rest of Europe
Trump's America, North Korea and Russia
And the sleeping giant, China
This country is going to have a general election soon
Would you rather be red than dead?
Do you want to live like a Russian or a North Korean?
Do you think Donald Trump has got it right in America?
I think he's a lot smarter than we thought
Is being a surrogate country to America really a choice?
Could we vote Jeremy Corbyn in and opt out of everything?
I don't think we can afford to do that
We would put our whole existence in jeopardy
Whilst Corbyn is a likeable idealist
I think he's a slate short of a roof
If he thinks he's capable of running this country
With no nuclear weapons and no American big brother
It will be interesting to see who gets elected to parliament

Andrew Aldred

The Latest Thing

Here she is on MTV
She's the latest thing to break
She's got a load of videos on the internet
She plays festivals all over Europe
She can sing a bit and write songs
She's collaborated with some big names
God knows I wish her luck
My girlfriend wants to go and see her show
She's not really my sort of thing
She's far too young
And I'm not down with the kids
Everyone I liked in music died
Or they're sat next to a swimming pool
In a hotel somewhere in the sun
She's the new breaking act
I'll keep my eye out for her
And see how long she lasts

There's Light at the End of the Tunnel

The Imperfect Poet

I'm something of an imperfect poet
I don't stand on a soapbox in my hometown
Bellowing out crap trying to sell a pile of books
I suppose you disagree with me over a lot of issues
Although on others I hope there's some consensus
The only reason I've got any money
Is because I don't spend it as quickly as everybody else
Some might think I'm a bit of a miser
But I'm very far removed from being a millionaire
If I had some money I'd buy a better car
And some more fashionable, newer clothes
I provide a lot of problems and very few solutions
With what I write in my books
My language isn't romantic or eloquent
But most people know what I mean
I'll never be as well respected as Philip Larkin
And I'll never sell as well as Leonard Cohen
Being an imperfect poet is where my strength lies

Andrew Aldred

License to be Irresponsible

They've given Donald Trump a license
To do what the hell he wants in America
I'm scared they'll give Jeremy Corbyn the same
At least the French voted Macron to power
And the nationalist party has faded into the background
If you're going to vote don't think the impossible
Don't vote for somebody as a novelty or a joke
What happens when they've got into power?
The public only has to get rid of them again
And it's difficult to get back to where you were before
Because your country has lost so much ground
What's the point in nationalising the railways?
Why give everyone education for free?
Does Jeremy Corbyn want to pay my mortgage as well?
We're already going to owe the EU fifty billion pounds
So let's just spend another fifty billion
To get out of debt? Don't make me laugh!
If you're going to tell me a fairy tale
At least make it somehow plausible
Get the clowns out and send the labour party in!

There's Light at the End of the Tunnel

1.7 Trillion

Almost two trillion pounds sterling
That's the national debt these days
Or so I heard on radio two
That's a hundred and fifty thousand pounds
For every man, woman and child in this country
If I have got my sums right
That's at least three year's wages
If everyone had a good job
I'm watching the political parties tonight
Harping on about social care
Saying the NHS needs more money
That's all very well, but listen
What do we really own in this country?
If everyone owes a hundred and fifty thousand pounds
We need a twenty-year plan
To sort out the national debt
We have to live within our means
And save whatever we can for our children
And hope whoever we owe the money to
Doesn't walk in and take over our country
Nobody talks about it any more
But we owe someone some serious money

Andrew Aldred

Out-trumped

Donald Trump has sacked one too many people
In his recent re-shuffle at the White House
He's had one too many dealings with the Russians
Everything will start to come to light
Everyone is asking questions and wanting answers
All Donald Trump can call it is a witch-hunt
But why do people hunt witches down and kill them?
Only because they've had enough of being persecuted themselves
Donald Trump is going to struggle to employ anyone
Because they won't keep their job long
They're going to be asked to conceal the truth
And then be made the fall-guy for the president
When is he going to get his come-uppance?
It won't be much longer by the looks of things

There's Light at the End of the Tunnel

Potentially failed Business

They are over-eager to help you
Selling vape liquids like quack doctors
Irresponsible and money-grabbing
We had a conversation with one of them
His supplier bought a machine from China
But there was a part missing
And they can't get the vape liquids
Then they got busted by trading standards
For having illegal stock on display
Why couldn't they get rid of it?
They're all too gung-ho for my liking
The other shops are on top of everything
Their vape liquids and e-cigs are legal
And everything else has been disposed of
Since the changes in the law
They've got the best situation in Farnworth
But they're the worst in terms of management
And they're on the way to being a failed business

Andrew Aldred

Re-incarnation of Margaret Thatcher

Theresa May is in charge of government now
And there's already a huge drive towards monetary policy
My girlfriend is going to get her benefits cut
She's had a heart attack a year ago
And tried to get a job all her life
Without a lot of success
She's a lovely person with a crippling illness
We're going to have less money than we had
They're going to reduce the deficit
By taking money off people who have little enough
It's socially and morally wrong
But everyone is going to have to pay
To get the deficit down to an acceptable level
There's going to be a two-tier society
Everyone is going to be squeezed
Those of us in good jobs will feel it less
Theresa May will get in at the next election
It's the nineteen eighties all over again
Is Theresa May a reincarnation of Margaret Thatcher
She's inherited a similar social situation
In an economically and socially unstable country

There's Light at the End of the Tunnel

Manchester Bombing

Where do we breed all these terrorists?
Is this the best thing that a twenty-two-year old can do?
To blow himself and twenty-two people up?
Anyone should be worth better than that
He has allowed himself to be radicalised
And filled with hatred for all those around him
By religious bigots who are worse people than himself
Too cowardly to commit the act they perpetrated
We need to pool our communities together
To protect people from being radicalised
To make people part of something in the community
Whether it be family, religion or mental health
Separate communities with pockets of terrorism are no good
And we need to flush them out of our society
To convert people's energy into some useful effort
And promote social inclusion instead of radicalisation

Andrew Aldred

Who should I vote for?

I watched them all on television last night
All of the political parties in one debate
One to the left of centre and one to the right
One for Scotland and one for Wales
One just heckling everyone and saying nothing
One skinhead in a suit and one well-meant environmentalist
All stood in a room and trying to deny each other the right to speak
And somehow I have to decide who to elect out of this rabble
I want my vote to count so it has to be labour or conservative
I want to retain my benefits and I want my girlfriend to retain hers
But I also want to vote for the good of the country
To reduce the national deficit and not to waste money
Should I vote for personal gain and labour?
Or make the sacrifice and vote conservative?
I've made my choice and I hope you've made yours
I await the result of the election with anxious anticipation!

There's Light at the End of the Tunnel

Soul in Torment

My life has been one series of bad events
Coupled with an awful coincidence of health problems
It's no wonder I've ended up being paranoid
Nothing ever goes right for very long in my life
I'm just not that lucky person, rather the opposite
I've always felt a bit like Job in the bible
Everything is a continual test of my faith
And believe me I've faltered more than once
Life is a continual battle between myself and my demons
Cancer, heart attack and all manner of health problems
Sometimes I really need some relief from life
At least I've got a house of my own now
A place of rest and refuge from everyone
Paranoia is the worst illness that I've got
I'm a soul in torment ruled by fear sometimes!

Andrew Aldred

Us This Year

We've been through a hell of a lot recently
She's been by my side through cancer
And all the way through my recovery
We're working hard to try to improve our health
Not to drink or smoke. She's trying to lose weight
We're almost able to relax again
It's only austerity that we struggle with
Settling into our new life. Together most of the time
But able to have our own space if we want it
Keeping on top of things in our separate houses
Looking after our grandson and her mother
I'm truly proud of what we have achieved
We've found a new lease of life together
And we really couldn't have done it without each other

There's Light at the End of the Tunnel

Jeremy Corbyn Versus Theresa May

They were both on television promoting their politics
Both giving good, constructive answers to difficult questions
She was lacking on social policy and monetarism
He collapsed on his lack of willingness to defend the country
In the event of a nuclear attack. Would he press the button?
Only if we were struck first and maybe not even then
These are both gigantic failings in policy and personality
There hasn't been a lot of money put into public services recently
There aren't as many police and nurse's pay hasn't risen
Do Mr Corbyn's sums add up? Could he make things better?
Could we really take all the money off the super-rich?
Can we rely on corporation tax as much as Corbyn says?
Or is he going to force companies to close down
With his milestone ten pounds minimum wage?
If Theresa May gets in I hope her social policy gets better
If Jeremy Corbyn gets in I hope they don't bomb us!

Andrew Aldred

2017 Election

Jeremy Corbyn expects Theresa May to resign
Even though she's just formed a new government
Labour has done well but it's not a victory
The result represents a divided society
People that think they are owed a better standard of living
And people that don't or are satisfied with their lot
The monetary policy of the conservatives has gone far enough
There needs to be more money for the inner cities
There needs to be agreement over Brexit
Politicians need to co-operate with each other
Everyone needs to stop shouting shit and get on
The country needs some good decisions now
You can't run a government by sabotage or ignorance
We are a democracy and the vote represents just that

There's Light at the End of the Tunnel

Slowing Down

Love used to be all about sex
Drinking, mad passion and blatant sexuality
I remember being called a fornicator in Manchester City centre
By a bible-bashing man in an old suit
Sat on Piccadilly gardens next to café Nero
I had to realise I was slowing down
And she did as well. We got so unhealthy.
It took us a divorce and a year apart
To realise we were better off together
To realise just how much we have in common
Huge experience of mental illness and poverty
All the time spent as friends before the relationship
The educational qualifications and the effort to get on
The jobs we shared and the friends and family
The loneliness we experienced without each other
Our love is for all those around us now
We've both had our fling and we're settling down together

www.ingramcontent.com/pod-product-compliance
Ingram Content Group UK Ltd.
Pitfield, Milton Keynes, MK11 3LW, UK
UKHW041413180426
11947UKWH00007B/110